DR. HUSSEIN KANDIL

The Male

Pearls of Hope in Male Infertility

This book was professionally typeset on Reedsy.
Find out more at reedsy.com

"To my family, all my mentors and teachers, and most importantly, my very precious patients who were my greatest teacher, and to whom I dedicate this humble book, hoping I pay back a bit of what you have given me."

*"The continuity of human race is a tun-
nel, and on one side is Men's Health."*

Hussein Kandil, MBBCh, FACS

Contents

Preface

Male infertility is defined as inability of the male to induce pregnancy, and accounts for 50% of infertility cases. Recently, research communities have implemented numerous task forces to investigate etiologies and more importantly offer guidelines for the management of male infertility. With a rising incidence affecting the developed and developing countries altogether, the need for proper identification of various hazards and risk factors for male factor infertility remains crucial.

Male infertility is a complex disorder with multi-factorial etiologies and may come forth with different presentations. Despite all this, our present enlightenment is honorably progressing, and our current knowledge surmounts the mediocrity and darkness overwhelming this condition in the past.

The taboos and social complexities revolving against discussing male reproduction was a major obstacle for data collection, unfortunately contributing to the deterioration in research capacity and ultimately lack of proper and comprehensive understanding of male infertility in the past century.

The infertile couples go through a tough journey starting from the distressful situation discovering their sterility, to the frequent medical visits seeking one clinic after the other, and finally to the expensive medical tests and therapies craving for proper counseling and most importantly hope.

It is believed that with appropriate comprehension and careful guidance, great results could be achieved.

Infertile couples abide to pursuing information either through online web search, community journals or media related queries, seeking guidance and hunting for a chance, however this may unexpectedly lead them to the imprecise science, faulty information, inaccurate data and most seriously improper counseling and recommendation of using unsafe remedies. Here lies the importance of patient education, reading through the pages of this book will help patients expand their knowledge, establish better communication with their health care provider, become more actively involved in the decision making process, and ultimately empowering optimism during this agonizing journey.

This book is designed for infertile male patients as it draws light over this seemingly complicated and sensitive disorder, affecting the male in the core of his essence; his fertility.

The chapters within tackle various conditions predisposing to male sub-fertility or diseases linked to male sterility in a simplified, easy to read, and a comprehensive way. It portrays the milestones the patient usually goes through from diagnosis to management, implementing the latest updates in the field and using the most recent evidence based research and international guidelines. From my experience as a male infertility specialist and the inherited experience of my mentors ahead of me, one crucial lesson was learned, that patience remains the role model of this journey, which is sadly unbearable to many across the world, and that delivering hope can never succeed without adequate education and awareness, and here comes the essence of my book.

This book will navigate through various medical disorders related to male infertility in depth, simplified to be well digested by non-medical professionals, to help the patient know his next step, ask the right question to his health care provider, and prepare him self to what is lying ahead; giving no place for surprises and false hopes. Instead he will be able to reason with knowledge, avoid unnecessary waste of time and money on false information and faulty treatments.

Each segment of the book ends with a pearl of wisdom that offers a meaningful and insightful instruction to the reader, reiterating critical recommendations, expanding patient's awareness, and preparing him to pursue the next step.

At the end and as a reminder, the field of medicine concerned with male infertility remains evolving, and what is applicable today may become obsolete by the near future, and since schools of thought may vary among various professionals, the information gathered in this book may not reflect all concepts adopted worldwide, and doesn't represent the sole way of management of male infertility, yet it portrays a commonly used practice endorsed by many male infertility specialists worldwide. And since current scientific data are prone to omission by more contemporary and modern evidence based updates, it is strongly advised to maintain a contact with your health care provider who can offer an appropriate education and update to your knowledge abiding with the constantly evolving flow of scientific research and evidence-based medicine.

Kindly note that this book represents an educational tool and should not replace consulting your medical care provider, and any piece of information within this book should be discussed thoroughly with your physician.

I

Pearls of Knowledge

In order to understand the whereabouts of male infertility, highlighting the science behind the reproductive function remains crucial

Male Reproductive Physiology and Anatomy

The control of reproductive functions starts from the brain glands (the hypothalamus and pituitary gland) collectively known as the 'maestro'. They regulate many functions of the body, and reproduction is simply one of them. The process starts after secretion of specific set of hormones (Follicle Stimulating Hormone 'FSH', and Luteinizing Hormone 'LH') collectively known as the gonadotropins (GN's) that are delivered through the blood circulation to the testes where they play a pivotal role in human male reproduction.

Once GN's reach the testes, they act on specific type of cells stimulating them to grow and undergo maturation until they become mature sperms. They also act on a different type of cells within the testis, called the Leydig cells, signaling them to manufacture and secret the most important male reproductive hormone; Testosterone.

There is a control system that maintains balance and prevents exhaustion of the brain glands, called the feedback mechanism, which resembles the fridge thermostat used to stabilize temperature and hence prevents the extensive over-use of the machine. The same happens within our bodies, the brain glands senses the function of the testis namely sperm formation and testosterone secretion, and if adequate then GN's release into the blood circulation will slow down (Offering the brain glands a time for rest), yet if any disorder inflicts damage to testicular functions; immediate activation of the brain glands will take place, increasing the rate of release of gonadotropins, *as a call for rescue*, to support the threatened testis, aiming to enhance sperm formation and testosterone secretion back to normal.

Anatomy of the male reproductive tract is composed of the testis epididymis, vas deferens, seminal vesicles, prostate gland and the penis.

Our description of the anatomy of the male reproductive system will start from where the spermatic journey starts, the testis. The male has two testes, both situated in the scrotum, which has a lower temperature compared to the rest of the body, acting as a cooling system, and therefore offering a better milieu for the sperm forming machinery which normally requires lower temperatures. The testis is composed of densely packed tiny spaghetti like structures called the seminiferous tubules, within these tubules sperms are normally found. Also present is a group of sperm supporting cells called 'Sertoli cells'. They support, nourish and facilitate the growth and maturation of immature sperm cells until they become mature sperms. Finally, the Leydig cells, which are another group of cells located in between the seminiferous tubules and function as the main source of testosterone synthesis and secretion.

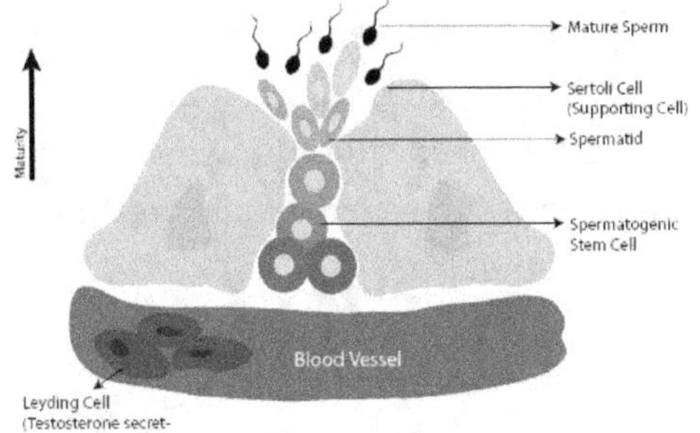

Sperm maturation cycle (Spermatogenesis)

Sperms once reach certain degree of maturation they pass from the testis towards the epididymis, a small organ surrounding on the back of the testis, where they acquire the function of motion and are rendered motile sperms.

A sperm is made of head (DNA chamber), neck (Source of energy), and a tail (Source of motion). Motility is achieved through a well-designed movement of the tail, which creates forward propelling thrust causing the sperm to move from the epididymis towards the storage glands (Seminal vesicle). The seminal vesicles are situated close to the urinary bladder and prostate gland, and secret a nourishing fluid (90% of the seminal volume) supporting the sperms through their journey.

At this point, the semen which is composed of sperms mixed up with seminal vesicle and prostatic fluids is ready for ejaculation, a process where the semen is forcibly passed through the penis and ultimately into the vagina.

In summary, the maestro; the brain glands secretes GN's into the bloodstream (FSH and LH), which stimulate the testes to manufacture sperms and secrete testosterone respectively. Sperms formed by the testis then pass to the epididymis for maturation then pass through the vas deferens for storage where they receive the nourishing secretions from the seminal vesicle and the prostate gland just prior to ejaculation, which is the forceful ejection of semen collectively from the male urethra to the exterior; in to the female genital tract.

Risk Factors and Causes of Male Infertility

Male infertility is a multifactorial disorder, and various risk factors play role in suppressing male fertility. Our daily life style involves hazardous exposures that negatively affect reproductive function. It is so difficult to encompass all possible risk factors and hazards, yet will sum up here the most common disorders causing male infertility.

Smoking:

Smoking is accused in wide range of medical disorders, and is a common preventable cause of many diseases. Recent trials have studied the causal connection between smoking and male fertility suppression and discovered that many deleterious particles are transferred through tobacco fumes into the testis and ultimately damage sperms; resulting in suppression of various sperm parameters and fertility potential. Smoking causes damage to the sperm DNA, which leads to deterioration of function and marked reduction in the sperm fertilizing capacity. Additionally, a study showed that sperm DNA abnormalities caused by smoking may be genetically transferred to the off springs of smokers. In some reports it is proven that smoking results in decline in testosterone levels adding to its negative effects on fertility.

Pearl of wisdom:

- *Quitting smoking is highly recommended not only for those who desire starting a family, but also to all population pursuing a healthy life.*

Alcohol:

Alcohol can impair human reproduction and results in reduction of male fertility at different levels. Some studies incriminated alcohol to cause testicular damage leading to reduction in testosterone secretion and diminution of sperm counts. Additionally it causes suppression of liver function; which is the source of elimination of many toxic materials in the body. When these toxic elements accumulate (due to liver malfunction) they result in deleterious effects on testicular function and ultimately affect sperm production. One additional adverse effect is the accumulation of the normally existing small concentrations of estrogens, resulting from reduced elimination by the defective liver, and therefore the build-up of estrogen associated with decline in testosterone are incriminated to negatively affect male reproduction and sexuality.

Pearl of wisdom:

- *Despite effects of alcohol are temporary yet chronic abuse may lead to long-term damage; so don't start now.*

Marijuana:

Tetrahydrocannabinol (THC), the medical term for the active ingredient of marijuana or referred to as 'pot'. Recent studies showed the detrimental effect of marijuana on male fertility. THC causes impairment in Leydig cell function (Cells responsible for testosterone formation and secretion). This results in major reduction in testosterone measurements; explaining the high incidence of low testosterone levels among marijuana addicts. It may also affect sperm production and function (Suppression in fertilizing capacity).

Pearl of wisdom*:*

- *THC addiction could be easily managed at specialized facilities, be honest and transparent while conveying to the health care provider your need for guidance and support, it only takes a single step.*

Obesity:

Male reproduction is violated by many conditions out of which obesity at the reproductive age. Over the last decade obesity has become an epidemic, with tremendous rise in prevalence, possibly as one of the major shortcomings of the modern life styles. This condition can be attributed to excessive consumption of processed food (High fat contents), empowering less physical activity and adapting a more sedentary life style. Aside from the commonly known diseases incriminated by obesity such as diabetes, high cholesterol levels, hypertension and heart disease, the deleterious effects on male reproduction could not be overlooked. Some studies have shown that testosterone levels may be reduced and estrogen levels are occasionally elevated among obese patients. On a different level, numerous studies have displayed the deleterious impact of obesity on the testis, causing major sperm defects and hence significant fertility suppression.

Pearl of wisdom:

- *Losing weight is considered as one major remedy to restore male fertility and sexuality, and its difficulty is out weighed by the significant positive impact on health and needless to say on male fertility.*

Testosterone Shots (T-Shots):

Every time we come across those heavily built and muscular athletes a question pops in to our minds, is it genuine or artificial?

Steroids, or exogenously administered testosterone shots (T-shots) are used for several indications, and whether used for medical purposes or as recreational performance enhancing drugs (Muscle building and repair) they have profound impact on male fertility. Indications make no difference when it comes to T-shot effects on male reproduction, they may render the male infertile. By the time a testosterone shot is administered, brain glands recognize it immediately, however it lacks the capacity to identify its source, whether it being from the testes (Endogenous) or simply an injection (Exogenous T-shot). As described previously, the brain glands act through the feedback mechanism, same as the fridge thermostat, so after receiving

T-shots, the brain glands will immediately shut down all gonadotropins (GN's) to the testes namely the LH and FSH (Being tricked thinking that this massive testosterone levels are coming from the testes), however this will ultimately result in marked reduction in the natural testosterone secretion from the testis (Endogenous) and eventually arrest in sperm production.

Pearl of wisdom:

- *For those considering using anabolic steroids (T-shots), building a family is more valuable and precious than building muscles.*
- *Be careful since messing with your hormones can be dangerous and may lead to uneventful outcomes.*
- *Evidence suggests an increasing incidence of hypogonadism (low testosterone levels) among males in their reproductive age and specifically males suffering from infertility, therefore it remains crucial to discuss with your physician alternative ways to boost your natural testosterone production, rather than receiving T- shots that can be damaging to fertility (At specific situations, T-shots are only given to patient declaring no desire of fertility preservation).*

Heat exposure:

The testis which is the prime male reproductive organ displays temperature sensitivity, and the inadvertent heat exposure may result in reduction in sperm quality and quantity; this explains why the testes are normally situated externally in the scrotum unlike the ovaries in females, escaping the relatively high core body temperature. Sources of heat exposure are multiple e.g.

heat emitted from laptops especially when placed over the thighs, frequent use of saunas, hot tubs and heated whirlpools, wearing tight pants and under garments and working close to heat source as in factories or in front of ovens.

Pearl of wisdom:

- *Stay away from heat, wear light loose underwear and avoid hot water exposure if you are planning to start a family.*

Radio-frequency:

Over the last decade, telecommunication has grown to occupy the frontier of modern technology, and has become a crucial mean of daily human communication (e.g. Cellular phones). This implicated daily exposure to the endless fields of radio-frequency and electromagnetic waves. Recently, surveys have shown increased rates of male infertility worldwide, and upon studying the underlying factors possibly explaining this un-precedented reduction of male fecundity; radio-frequency and electromagnetic waves (Emitted through cellular phones and other portable telecommunication devices) were listed among possible triggers. A study showed that radio-frequency waves may cause deterioration of sperm parameters. Unfortunately cellular phones are commonly placed into the trousers pocket (Making them in close proximity to the male gonads), negatively affecting fertility through exposing the testes to high power density cell phone radiation and hence causing deterioration in fertility.

Pearl of wisdom:

- *It is advisable to avoid increased exposure to radio-frequency electromagnetic fields by keeping cellular phones away from the testes.*

13

Genetic Diseases

Genes are the basic units of heredity, and are composed of the most fundamental structure of all organisms; the DNA. They exist in every cell of our body and are clustered together to form chromosomes. Each gene demands the body to perform a specific function e.g. color of the eyes, tissue growth or secretion of body fluids. Humans have 46 chromosomes, clustered in 23 pairs, 22 of which are dedicated for general body functions and therefore are common between males and females. One single pair determines the gender of the individual; hence based on those chromosomal patterns we get 46 (XX) and 46 (XY) for the females and males respectively.

Y chromosome dictates the masculine features and triggers the developing human embryo to become a male. In unfortunate circumstances some genetic errors involving either the number or the structure of the chromosomes may ensue and their manifestations depend on which chromosome is damaged. In the context of male infertility, many genetic syndromes are studied, yet will discuss here the more commonly encountered ones.

Pearl of wisdom:

- *Genetic testing for male infertility is a simple blood test that can be pricey with uncertain insurance coverage at different institutions worldwide.*
- *Not every laboratory can perform such testing, however specialized centers offering a wide range of genetic analysis exist nowadays.*
- *Karyotype is the genetic test that studies the number of your chromosome (normal male is '46XY'), Y-chromosome testing is the test that studies the integrity of the Y chromosome in cases of suspected damage e.g. micro-deletion.*

Klinefelter syndrome, 47 XXY (KS):

This rare genetic disorder affects only the male population, it occurs at incidence of 1 to 2 every 1000 males, with an onset of diagnosis at time of puberty. This syndrome is defined as the abnormal addition of one extra 'X' chromosome to the pre-existing 46 chromosomes, resulting into a total of 47 chromosomes '47 XXY'.

The extra 'X' chromosome triggers abnormalities in testicular formation, and ultimately loss of function of the testis, reaching the extent of total sperm absence in the ejaculate (Azoospermia). Additionally testosterone production may be reduced, and in some cases patients are usually managed through a life long testosterone therapy. Additionally, in KS estradiol levels may record higher levels, a condition that explains the enlarged breasts which is a common clinical feature, requiring estrogen lowering therapy.

With the help of modern sperm harvesting procedures (Also known as testicular biopsies) sperms can be successfully retrieved in number of patients and are subsequently used in assisted reproduction (Read below) fortunately offering KS patients the chance to father children.

Pearl of wisdom:

- *Genetic abnormality of Klinefelter syndrome may be transmitted to the male off springs and therefore genetic counseling is mandatory prior to any trial of conception (Sometimes cells from the embryos are retrieved and studied using a test called Pre-Implantation Genetic Diagnosis (PGD) to check for any possible inherited genetic abnormalities).*
- *Diagnosis of KS is crucial not only for its reproductive consequence but also to manage other sequelae associated with this disorder including cardiac, neurogenic and orthopedic anomalies.*
- *Management of KS may require time and effort so be patient and keep your hope alive, since sperm retrieval may be achievable with KS and fathering a child is never impossible; patience is virtue.*

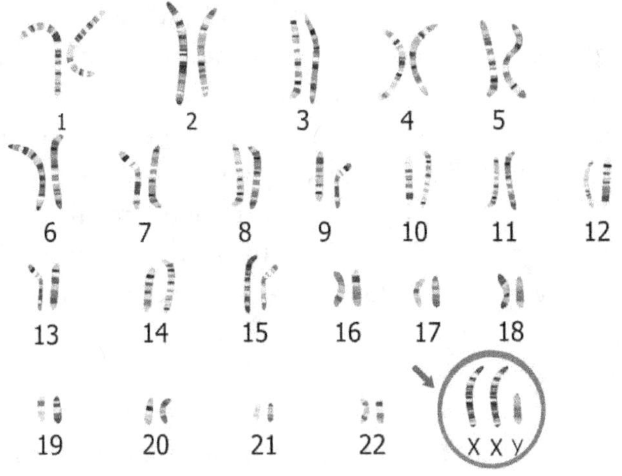

Klinefelter Syndrome 47 (XXY)

Y-Chromosome deletion:

Another genetic cause of male infertility is attributed to abnormality in the structure of the Y chromosome that normally triggers the developing embryo to become a male. Early in the process of development and in unfortunate circumstances, the Y chromosome is damaged and the male ends up with a dysfunctional Y chromosome, resulting in small defective testes, severely diminished number of sperms to the extent of total absence of sperms, and occasionally reduction of testosterone secretion from the testis, ultimately resulting in infertility and sexual dysfunction. Though this disorder hinders sperm production, occasionally small areas in the testis are spared, and can still produce scant number of sperms, yet are not enough to reach out and appear in the ejaculate. Therefore, when Y chromosome micro-deletion is diagnosed (Using genetic testing), the physician may advice to perform a microsurgical testicular biopsy (if sperms are not found in the ejaculate), offering a fairly decent success rate of sperm retrieval and ultimately using those sperms in assisted reproduction. It is noteworthy that location of the damage (Or micro-deletion) on the Y chromosome can predict the possibility of successful sperm recovery (Read below).

Pearl of wisdom:

- *Discuss with the infertility specialist the type of deletion on the Y-chromosome, and be informed that success rates of sperm retrieval can reach up to 40% in experienced hands.*

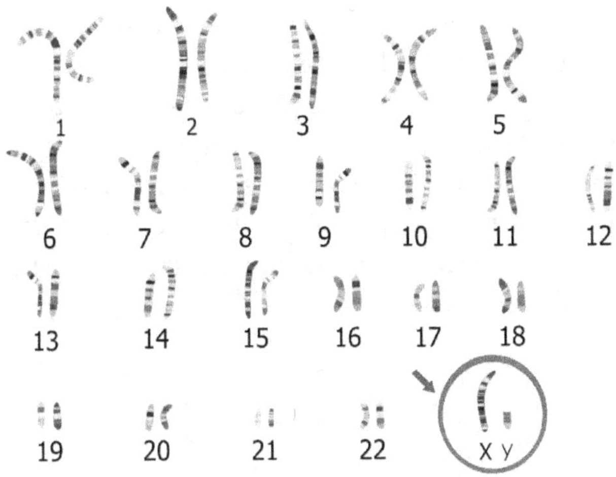

Y chromosome micro–deletion

Absence of the vas deferens:

The vas deferens is a tube like structure connecting the testes to the ejaculatory duct, which is the final station before the emission of semen during ejaculation. In unfortunate situations genetic errors (Or referred to as 'mutations') occur in the gene called 'Cystic Fibrosis Trans–membrane conductance Regulator gene (CFTR)' on chromosome number 7, causing a serious disease called 'cystic fibrosis', which can affect the digestive, respiratory, endocrine and reproductive systems. Reproductive traits of the disease include absence of the vas deferens on one or both sides of the body; causing blockage to the sperm pathways without affecting the actual sperm formation process inside the testes. When only one copy of the gene is damaged in a male patient, the person is rendered a carrier of the disease and is otherwise healthy (Other than having the vas deferens absent). It is recommended that couples with either a personal or close family history of cystic fibrosis be tested, the female partner should be also tested for possible concurrent mutation of the same gene, and incase both partners have mutations of the CFTR gene, their off springs will have high probability acquiring 'cystic fibrosis disease' and the couples should be counseled about this possible risk.

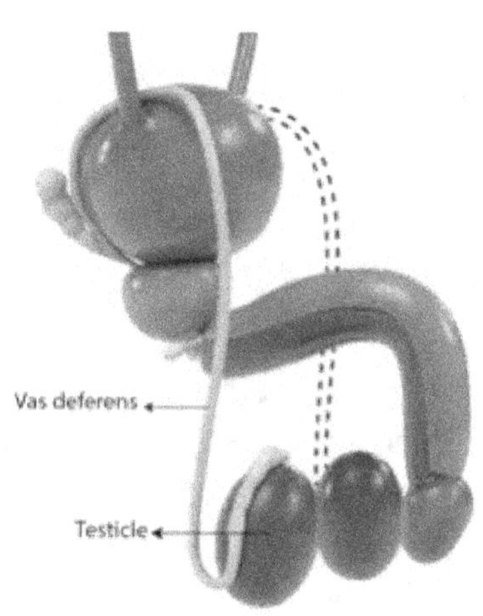

Illustration showing absence of one vas deferens

Pearl of wisdom:

- *Though sperms are lacking in the ejaculate of patients with absent vas deferens; the sperm formation is completely normal, and fathering a child will be through harvesting sperms from the testis (Biopsy) and using those retrieved sperms in assisted reproduction, of course after performing a genetic test to the female partner. Hence, absence of the vas deferens doesn't imply absolute infertility.*

Low Testosterone (Hypogonadism)

Testicular function includes testosterone secretion and sperm formation. Low testosterone or the medical term commonly used 'Hypogonadism' is diagnosed when any of those functions is hindered, but this term is commonly attributed to states of testosterone deficiency. As mentioned previously in the physiology of male reproduction, the brain glands (Hypothalamus and pituitary glands) release the first signal to testosterone secretion through the Luteinizing Hormone (LH), conveying the message to the testes; and if properly functioning, each testis obeys and responds by secreting testosterone hormone from group of specialized cells called leydig cells. Many disease conditions can affect this orchestral harmony (Diseases of the brain glands or diseases involving the testes). Testosterone has many functions including (but not limited to) the following:

- Supports the machinery of sperm formation inside the testes.
- Essential for most of spermatic functions including the integrity of sperm DNA, motility and fertilizing capacity.
- Plays an important role in male sexuality and libido (sexual drive).
- Essential for penile growth and health, making it crucial for

sexual and erectile function.
- Enhances the metabolic functions of the body and augment fat burning.
- Being an anabolic steroid, it enhances muscular growth and repair.
- Maintains bone growth and integrity.

Testosterone exists in two different forms: bound (Inactive) and bioavailable testosterone (Active). When diagnosed with low testosterone level, your physician will check your LH to assess the function of the brain glands. Low testosterone associated with low LH is suggestive of brain gland anomaly (Dysfunctional brain glands are incapable of secreting enough LH to stimulate the testes to secrete testosterone). On the other hand, low testosterone measurement associated with high levels of LH is suggestive of testicular failure (The brain glands are reacting by releasing more LH to support the deteriorating testes, aiming to improve the low testosterone level). It is not surprising that sperm formation (Quantity and quality) is dramatically reduced in face of low testosterone level, and treating male infertility is never successful without proper hormonal evaluation and correction of underlying testosterone deficiency. In addition to the impact of low testosterone on fertility, males may also convey sexual complaints, including low sexual drive (Libido), weak erections (Erectile dysfunction), and abnormal or weak ejaculations.

Pearl of wisdom:

- _Hormonal testing should be performed between 8am and 11am (normally hormonal secretion declines afterwards coinciding_ *with the human biological clock).*

- *Insurance coverage varies from one company to other (Hormonal tests can be pricey) so check with your insurance agent prior to testing.*
- *It is preferable and more accurate to calculate the bioavailable testosterone instead of only measuring the total testosterone.*
- *Associated sexual dysfunction symptoms with infertility may predict an underlying hormonal abnormality (Caused by low level of testosterone).*
- *Symptoms of low testosterone may resemble those of depression, so have your testosterone checked when in doubt of mood disorder.*
- *Some labs measure the free testosterone which is less informative than measuring the bioavailable testosterone.*

Varicocele

As with any organ in the body, the testis has it is own blood supply; the arteries delivering clean blood from the heart to the testis and the veins pumping wasteful blood back to the heart for cleansing. Occasionally the valves in the testicular veins (Normally present to prevent back flow of blood) are damaged, and after some time cause enlargement and swelling of those veins lying around the testes a condition also known as *Varicocele.* This unfortunate phenomenon disturbs the testicular milieu by transmitting the blood temperature (i.e., 37.2 degrees C) to the testis (Normally the testicular temperature is lower than the core body temperature to allow for normal sperm production). Warming of the testes threatens sperm formation and may lead to reduction in testicular size. The dysfunctional veins release toxins that eventually cause direct damage to the sperm forming cells. Varicoceles are considered a common cause of reversible infertility in males, and may be incriminated in few studies to lower testosterone hormone. Predisposing factors for varicoceles are prolonged standing, sitting and pressure (Weight lifting).

Pearl of wisdom:

- *To avoid varicocele try to have enough rest following periods of exhaustion and prolonged standing, so whenever feasible lay down and have your lower extremities raised over a pillow.*
- *Difference in the size of both testes in adolescents may be an alarming sign of varicoceles that warrants evaluation and treatment.*

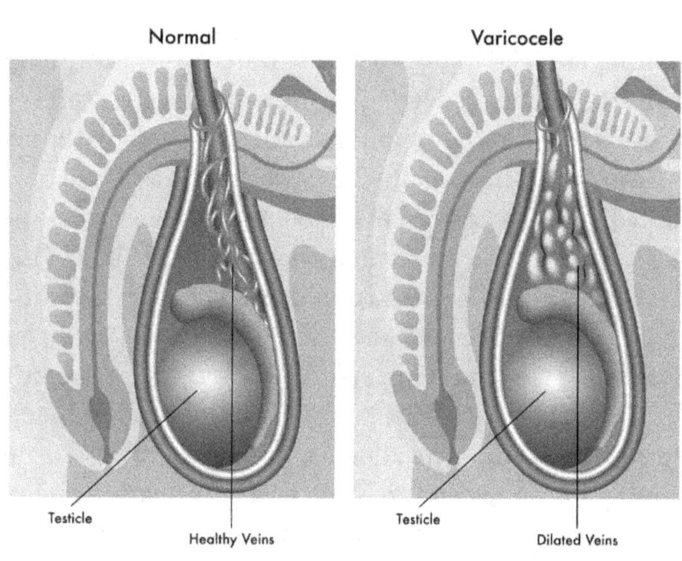

Varicocele

Undescended Testis

Many parents of male children panic when fail to identify one or both testes in the scrotum. Yes, the testes may fail to descend into their normal position and become stuck in abnormal locations inside the body, causing serious damage and loss of function (Testosterone secretion and sperm formation). Being stuck inside the body exposes the testis to the deleterious effect of the relatively high core body temperature, causing the testis to shrink and lose most of its volume, and with time this damage renders the male infertile.

Pearl of wisdom:

- *Parents should be vigilant inspecting the genitalia of their male off-springs while changing their diapers.*
- *The earlier the testis is brought back into the scrotum; the higher the chance of recovery and better prognosis salvaging future fertility.*

Testicular Inflammation

Inflammation of the testis causes disruption of the testicular tissues, where suddenly millions of inflammatory cells permeate into the testis and epididymis, releasing many toxic materials that damage the cell lines responsible for sperm formation. *Mumps virus* is one serious viral infection that inflicts children, and despite the decline of incidence following the widespread vaccination, it remains a serious disease. Mumps virus attacks the parotid glands and may occasionally involve and cause severe damage to the testes, complicating significant drop in sperm counts, and subsequently male infertility.

Pearl of wisdom:

- *Vaccination is mandatory when it comes to protecting against mumps and its related consequences.*
- *Consult an urgent care facility when suspecting testicular infection (Sudden testicular swelling associated with pain and fever).*

Disorders of Ejaculation

Ejaculation is the forceful emission of seminal fluid containing the sperms and secretions from the male reproductive glands through the urethra at the time of climax or male orgasm. During ejaculation the urinary bladder becomes firmly closed to prevent the backward migration of the seminal fluid into the urinary bladder (a disorder known as retrograde ejaculation). The forceful emission is necessary to propel the semen (Containing the sperms) deep in to the vagina, hence any disease states interfering with normal ejaculation may lead to infertility. Several conditions are incriminated to induce ejaculatory dysfunction. Possible scenarios include conditions that affect the bladder integrity e.g. following surgical removal of an enlarged prostate e.g. prostate or bladder surgeries, consequently the bladder will fail to close during ejaculation, leading to retrograde emission of the semen backwards into the urinary bladder. Other conditions affecting normal ejaculation include an adverse effect of a class of medications called 'alpha blockers' (Used to treat enlarged prostates), such medication may interfere with the innervation controlling ejaculation, complicating failure of seminal emission (Anejaculation) and hence infertility (Read below about management of ejaculatory dysfunction). On the other hand, some people may complain of either rapid or delayed ejaculation. Rapid ejaculation is commonly related to psychologic stress and hence is more experienced at the end of the day more than in morning times and on weekdays more than on weekends which are obviously periods where higher levels of stress are encountered. Delayed ejaculation is mostly attributed to neurologic/psychological causes. For instance, diabetic patients who suffer one of the common diabetic complications, being nerve damage, same as with any other nerve diseases, can experience failure of the ejaculatory mechanism due to damaged nerves. That being said, delayed ejaculation is a common side effect of anti-depressant medications, especially if taken in high doses.

Pearl of wisdom:

- *Alpha blockers are the standard therapy for enlarged prostates, and their paralyzing effect on the male glands is reversible, in other words; once the medication is stopped one should expect return of ejaculation.*
- *Patients with disordered ejaculation may still have normal sperm formation.*
- *Whether you suffer from a rapid or delayed ejaculation, treatments are available, so be advised to share this valuable piece of information with your doctor.*

II

What to Expect on the First Medical Consultation

The visit with the healthcare provider is very critical, so being prepared for such encounter will offer significant added value, being able to ask the right question and be prepared to align with the instructions offered to implement successful therapeutic roadmap.

Discussing Future Road Map and Patient's Critical Questions

At the end of the initial appointment with your infertility specialist, you will be asked to perform basic tests for male infertility including blood and sperm test (Read below about each test requested for fertility assessment), and upon the follow-up visit, the infertility specialist will discuss your results with you, going through each finding. It is not uncommon to have abnormal results, and it is your physician's duty to transmit all relevant information on how to manage each abnormalities. Occasionally you will be requested to repeat tests to confirm unusual results. At this point, your infertility specialist must be ready to make a preliminary diagnosis, and offer possible explanation behind your condition, however in some rare instances when basic evaluation returns equivocal; further advanced testing is required (Read below on advanced testing for fertility assessment). Now your therapeutic plan is ready for outline, clarified in a step-by-step fashion. It is not uncommon to receive more than one therapy at the same time based on your condition (Male infertility can be multifactorial and hence requires more than one treatment concurrently). If further testing appears necessary, your physician may postpone treatment until results are back one more time. Make sure you comprehend your physician's overview of your condition as this will help set your expectations on an appropriate scale. Go back through the therapeutic plan word by word with your physician, ask for further instructions related to your prescription including dosage, mode of administration, duration of therapy, possible interactions with other ongoing treatments, possible side effects and how to deal with missed or skipped doses. If needed convey your worry to your health care provider who must be ready to deal with your anxiety and properly address your concerns (That's normal so don't get embarrassed). You will be scheduled for a third return appointment for evaluation following therapy (Or if further testing was required you will need to return back to receive your therapeutic plan). Hormonal abnormalities require very delicate hormonal treatment that can be administered via oral route (Pills) or injections, and this may require delicate monitoring and accurate interval between dosages. Make sure to learn how to interact with your physician in cases of inadvertent occurrence of adverse events related to your therapy e.g. allergies. Other treatments may include antioxidants and food supplements that have recently gained some interest in the management of male infertility (Not fully accredited yet by international medical committees), antibiotics incases of infections (Check your allergy status), anti-inflammatory medications for genital inflammations (Patients with stomach problems should be cautious as these medications can hurt their stomach and cause ulcers). Finally, your wife will be asked to schedule an appointment with her gynecologist to evaluate her fertility status and rule out any possible female factor of infertility (Remember it is a teamwork).

Pearl of wisdom:

- *Abnormal test results are no reason for panic since many of them are correctable; so be optimistic.*
- *Inquire about alternative medications (it is common that some medicines can get cut off from the market).*
- *Many clinics help stop smoking and treat alcohol addiction; simply ask your physician to schedule an appointment for you.*
- *If desired, convey your interest in reading and learning more about your condition, your physician can supply you with the most suitable, accurate and up to date information resources.*

Assessment and Examination

Deciding to seek medical care is the first step towards therapy. Upon scheduling an appointment note that your physician is preferably an infertility specialist. Urologists are the ideal health care providers concerning male infertility, being well trained to deal with various male reproductive disorders (Medically and surgically). During years of urology residency training and post-graduate fellowships, the trainees go through intensive training and workshops in andrology, which is the field of urology that treats male infertility and sexual dysfunction. Before your scheduled visit prepare all previous medical records, and research your family history. Be aware that your physician may start posing relevant questions, starting by general inquiries to assess your overall health, then dwelling progressively to assess your fertility status, including but not limited to history of previous conceptions or abortions, sexual life, exposure to certain risk factors, relevant personal background or family history suggestive of ongoing genetic dysfunction, pharmaco-logical history e.g. intake of suspicious medications or hor-mones that can induce fertility suppression, previous surgeries with potential impact on fertility, spouse's medical condition including age, general health, menstrual cycle, and previous fertility evaluation and finally the contact of her gynecologist for establishing a teamwork communication. At this point and while responding to your physician's inquiries, be advised to respond with caution, for every answer has its value. Don't hesitate to ask your physician to rephrase any question again, for sometimes questions can sound complicated and may need further elaboration. If you have any relevant information in mind, and despite you are not being specifically asked about; don't hesitate to share them with your physician. Be advised to present to your physician all relevant previous tests e.g. previous blood or sperm tests, previous x-rays or reports of previous surgeries or hospitalizations. At some point the physician will offer to perform a comprehensive medical examination, which has two main parts, the first that evaluates the whole body and is called the general exam; this identifies the non genital signs of diseases that may contribute to infertility. Then will follow the detailed and comprehensive urologic exam that focuses on the genital examination, assessing the testicular shape, size, and the structures passing to and from them. Other genital exam includes the presence of worrisome lesions or abnormalities on the penis that warrant further testing. Examination also includes examining the prostate gland, which is done through a rectal test; this test assesses the size and the shape of the prostate gland and checks for unusual findings that could explain fertility suppression and hence warranting further testing.

Pearl of wisdom:

- *Be transparent with your physician and make extra effort to answer all questions in details.*
- *The physician who is under oath is there to help you and to*

protect your privacy, so feel free to address any issue that concerns you even if it feels so personal and private.

- Ask your infertility specialist to set your expectations.
- If desired, the presence of your spouse with you will help to ascertain her inquiries and concerns too.
- Expect that you will be requested to perform medical tests and will once again have to meet with your infertility specialist to discuss results and start planning your treatment plan.

III

Basic Evaluation of Male Infertility

The basic evaluation of the male reproductive function is considered mandatory, of course, keeping in mind the financial burden that may be laid upon the patient himself, however, whenever possible, these tests will offer significant level of understanding when it comes to the male fertility status, and may help differentiating between the ambitious causes of male infertility.

Semen Analysis

Though inconvenient and lacks accuracy, this test remains a vital when it comes to male fertility. Despite the fact that results may vary between different labs, and even along two different points of time (Which is a common finding among all males), semen analysis is still considered a standard test commonly used to test male fertility, and its role in the management and follow up remains pivotal. Examining sperms is critical and is dependent on the examiner's experience in most of available labs, and hence the subjective experience remains crucial when it comes to examining semen samples. Based on the current international guidelines; patient should perform at least two semen testing preferably at different institutions and at least two weeks apart. Once scheduled for a semen test, be instructed to abstain from ejaculating for three to five consecutive days (not more and not less), shorter periods of abstinence result in lower counts than actually present, and longer periods of abstinence may yield sperms with poor quality. Usually the test is performed in specialized centers that are well prepared and private enough to host such examination. Once ready, you will be handled a sterile collection cup in which you will be asked to ejaculate after masturbation. Make sure you collect all the ejaculated semen and avoid spillage.

Normally each drop of the semen may have millions of sperms and though loss of a single drop may seem trivial, yet its impact on accuracy of the test remains significant. If you fail to perform the test for its inconvenience, be advised to discuss with your physician the possibility of performing the test at your convenient location, and hence you will be given a specialized collection kit which can preserve the viability of the sample until its delivery back to the lab. A basic sperm test quantifies the volume of the ejaculated liquid, the number of the sperms in each one milliliter of the semen (concentration), the number of sperms with normal and abnormal motility and morphology and finally the number of unusual cells if present e.g. white blood cells (WBCs) that signifies the presence of inflammation and possible infection. Reading and interpreting result of a sperm test requires studying more than one semen sample since results may vary (as mentioned earlier). *In some instances, when sperm counts are very low (concentration below 5 million/ml), your infertility specialist may recommend sperm banking (Freezing of the sample) during the time of semen analysis, and to perform sperm banking you will be instructed to deliver more than one semen sample at different times to store more numbers of sperms.* Sperm banking by freezing is now a widespread practice by most of reproductive laboratories, and despite the preference of using a freshly obtained sperms, some studies show that stored sperms (Frozen) can still give good results as compared to fresh sperms.

Pearl of wisdom:

- *When asked to perform a semen test, try to perform two testings (instead of only one) at two different labs, and seek a reputable center since it depends on the experience of the examiner.*

- *In some instances the anxiety and stress are capable of hindering patient's erection, and therefore the test can become troublesome and eventually gets cancelled.*
- *Incases of inadvertent failure of inducing or maintaining an erection during the test, be advised to convey this to your physician who will prescribe you medications that supports a quick and strong erection.*
- *Avoid performing semen analysis at times of febrile illnesses as this may interfere with the accuracy of the test.*

Hormonal Evaluation

Hormonal abnormalities are potentially reversible causes of male sub-fertility and proper evaluation remains important aspect in the management of males presenting to a fertility clinic. Numerous hormones are enlisted for evaluation, however will discuss the most commonly used in the current clinical practice.

Gonadotropins (GN's):

Luteinizing Hormone (LH) and Follicle Stimulating Hormone (FSH), both hormones are secreted from the brain glands (the maestro as previously explained), they target the gonads in both genders (testes and ovaries). In the males LH interacts with the leydig cells of the testes triggering secretion of testosterone. On the other hand FSH interacts with another group of cells (Sertoli cells) that support sperm formation. Deficiency of gonadotropins leads to suppression of sperm formation and reduced testosterone levels. Low GN's may result from diseases affecting the brain glands (pituitary gland and hypothalamus). Those conditions may be congenital or acquired. In congenital disorders patients usually present with delayed puberty, lack of sexual development and ultimately infertility. In acquired diseases, patients may present with progressively declining testosterone levels, lowered sexual potency and libido (Sexual drive) and low sperm counts leading to infertility. Possible causes for acquired diseases include intake of exogenous anabolic steroids (Testosterone shots), chronic illness, head injury, chemotherapy, etc. On the other hand, High levels of GN's is commonly encountered when the testes fails to function properly i.e. failure of testosterone secretion and reduced sperm production, apparently any of these conditions seems to alarm the brain glands (Pituitary glands and hypothalamus) which respond by an increasing GN's secretion (Remember the thermostat example mentioned in earlier chapters).

Pearl of wisdom:

- *GN's release from brain glands is increased in response to dysfunction of the testes (Brain gland's rescue plan).*
- *High levels of FSH maybe associated with disorders of sperm formation in the testes, however normal levels cannot exclude testicular disorder.*
- *Specific forms of therapy raise testosterone levels through raising LH levels from the brain glands.*

Testosterone (Androgens):

Testosterone is probably the most popularly known among all hormones. Around 95% of circulating testosterone is secreted from the testes, and only smaller amounts are produced by the adrenal gland. Testosterone secretion in males starts at puberty when the testes receive an order from the brain to commence their activity. It plays central role in the development of male secondary sexual characteristics such as increase in hair growth, increase of muscle mass, deepening of the voice, coarsening of the skin and enlargement of the penis. It is also responsible for the process of sperm formation and maturation. Testosterone production is highest at the earlier hours of the day and starts to decline afterwards. Younger age population (Age between 20-30) has higher levels compared to older population where levels tend to decline.

Pearl of wisdom:

- *Be advised that the best time to test your testosterone hormone is early in the morning between 8am to 11am; corresponding with the time of higher physiologic levels (fasting is not required prior to measuring testosterone unless your investigation also includes other tests that require fasting e.g. cholesterol or blood sugar).*
- *Testing testosterone may require measuring other molecules to calculate the bioavailable testosterone, which assesses the concentration of the biologically active testosterone in your body.*
- *Bioavailable testosterone measurement is more accurate than the commonly measured free testosterone.*
- *If total testosterone is normal but the bioavailable portion is low, treatment is still mandatory.*

Estradiol (Estrogen):

Though known to be a female reproductive hormone, estrogen

exists in males too, yet in much smaller concentrations. Sources of estrogens in the male body are either internal or external. Internal source is from the conversion of testosterone to estrogen in certain tissues e.g fatty tissues, but its level remains low, maintaining a very delicate ratio between both hormones. External sources are possibly from excessive ingestion of estrogen rich products e.g. some herbal products. Estradiol is required for selected physiological roles in male reproduction e.g. certain stages of sperm maturation, and in male sexuality e.g. libido. Occasionally estradiol levels are elevated beyond normal. The following are examples of conditions that can cause rise in estrogen levels, (Other causes do exist but the following are more commonly attributing disorders):

- Obesity (Increase in fat concentration): encouraging more testosterone to estrogen transformation
- Liver disease: resulting in defective elimination of estrogen from the body e.g. complications of excessive alcohol ingestion
- Excessive use of plastic products containing Bisphenol-A (BPA) especially when heated (BPA is a molecule that mimics estrogen role in the male body i.e. referred to as hormonal disrupter).
- Excessive ingestion of dietary products rich in estrogenic components (e.g. flax seeds).
- Klinefelter syndrome (read above in genetic disorders).

Though estrogen is required for basic physiological roles in male growth (e.g. bone growth), reproduction and sexuality, however excess levels especially when associated with low testosterone levels may attribute to reproductive dysfunction e.g. abnormal spermatic function, and hence reduced fertility.

Pearl of wisdom:

- *Incorporating estrogen to hormonal evaluation offers better understanding of your hormonal function.*
- *Ask your physician how to avoid excessive estrogen in your diet.*
- *Be advised to use Bisphenol–A (BPA) free plastic containers (As advised by few studies).*
- *Avoid using herbal remedies without consulting your health care provider on possible adverse effects.*

Prolactin:

Prolactin is another hormone secreted from the pituitary gland, and is known for its role in the females to produce milk during lactation. Other functions include supporting metabolism and regulation of immune system. Excess levels of prolactin can have detrimental effects on reproduction by inhibiting GN's secretion (LH and FSH), ultimately lowering testosterone secretion and reducing sperm counts. Prolactin is considered a stress hormone, meaning that stress can alter its concentration in the body, and therefore it is highly recommended to repeat the test when results are abnormal (especially in periods of stress). Prolactinoma, a benign tumor of the pituitary gland, and is a common cause of elevated prolactin levels and subsequently male infertility. Poor thyroid gland function may implicate rise in prolactin levels and therefore patients presenting with high prolactin may warrant thyroid hormonal testing. Some medications that block the effect of dopamine can cause detrimental elevations of prolactin.

Pearl of wisdom:

- *Be advised to share with your physician the list of your medications (Remember side effects of certain medications may cause prolactin elevation).*
- *Prior to prolactin testing be instructed to abstain from strenuous exercise or exposure to high levels of stress (Such conditions may alter your test results).*
- *When confronted with elevated prolactin your physician will request imaging to the brain (MRI of the pituitary gland) to rule out possible Prolactinoma.*

Metabolic testing:

Metabolic syndrome is a constellation of disorders that are linked together, of which the most commonly encountered are obesity, diabetes, high cholesterol and triglycerides (Collectively known as Dyslipidemia), and cardiovascular diseases. Recent studies have demonstrated connection between disorders of men's health (Male reproduction and sexual dysfunction) and metabolic syndrome. Obesity has many deleterious effects on male reproduction and sexual dysfunction, and is considered central feature of metabolic syndrome, it may implicate male infertility through several ways including increased conversion of testosterone into estrogens (as mentioned earlier), release of toxic products that harm sperm formation and finally the accumulation of fat at the thighs can raise temperature around the scrotum which ultimately hinders sperm formation. Diabetes may affect male fertility through lowering of testosterone production (Explaining the lower testosterone levels among some diabetics), finally it may damage the sperm DNA leading to deterioration of sperm function. There is evidence that dyslipidemia may also result in deliberate release of some toxins into the testicular microenvironment leading to damage to the sperm structure and deterioration of function.

Pearl of wisdom:

- *Healthy life style including diet monitoring and weight loss will protect against metabolic syndrome and hence prevent the inadvertent consequences on male fertility.*

IV

Advanced Testing of Male Infertility

In some situations, the advanced testing is required to help attain an additional level of clarity, especially when the basic testing doesn't yield enough information to proceed with a therapeutic plan.

Ultrasound Study

Occasionally a testicular ultrasound is requested which is a non-invasive, non-painful and non-physically challenging test. Ultrasound is a useful tool to assess male reproductive structures including the testis, epididymis, seminal vesicle and prostate gland. However, Doppler Ultrasound is another variant required to evaluate the blood vessels of the testis, including the arteries which are the main source of blood supply, and the veins which are the sources of varicoceles. Your physician will request an ultrasound when in doubt of structural abnormalities of the testis, like feeling a lump in your testis, swelling of your scrotum, discrepancy of testicular sizes and signs suggestive of infection. Whenever there is a suspicion of varicoceles or defective blood supply a Doppler ultrasound will be requested (also referred to as 'Duplex scan') to properly evaluate the blood flow to and from the testis.

Pearl of wisdom

- *Stay warm prior to performing a scrotal ultrasound, warmth cause the skin of the scrotum to relax and hence facilitate your examination.*

DNA Fragmentation Tests

The sperm is considered to be a messenger that transports the genetic material of the male i.e. the DNA which resides in the sperm head, delivering it to join the DNA within the female ovum (Thanks to the function of sperm motility) to create an embryo with a complete genetic structure. The Sperm DNA represents half the genetic material of the future embryo while DNA of the ovum represents the other half, and therefore when the sperm and ovum unite in the act of fertilization, a baby with a full number of chromosomes is created (46 chromosomes; 23 from the father and 23 from the mother). So it is clear why sperm DNA integrity is vital for fertilization and embryo formation. Having a normal semen test can still mask an underlying sperm dysfunction. DNA fragmentation test is valuable to assess sperm DNA integrity, and despite lack of definite guidelines to rationalize the use of DNA fragmentation tests in the management of male infertility, it has become a common practice among many infertility specialists. Factors implicated in sperm DNA damage may include increased age, smoking, varicocele, exposure to radiation, exposure to toxic environment, chemotherapy, metabolic syndrome, etc. Several assays varying in accuracy, availability and pricing are commercially available to study DNA integrity.

Pearl of wisdom

- *DNA fragmentation test is not a routine male fertility test, and is best indicated in the context of recurrent abortions or miscarriages, delayed pregnancy despite having a normal semen testing and unexplained infertility.*
- *Repeat the test after therapy to make sure your DNA integrity is improving, and hence sperms on the start line are healthy and ready to function.*

Genetic Testing

A genetic test is a blood test that evaluates the chromosomal structure and number. Male factor infertility can be attributed to genetic diseases, which are disorders caused by abnormalities in the structure or the number of certain chromosomes. Genetic tests are currently available worldwide, and though possibly considered pricey, they have become reputable and recommended in the context of male infertility. Other than diagnosing chromosomal aberrations incriminated as a cause of sterility, genetic tests are recommended to predict success of therapy, as with patients inflicted with Y-chromosome micro-deletions (Read earlier), the presence of a deletion of specific gene sites on the Y-chromosome (e.g. AZF a-b) are associated with severe testicular dysfunction and hence, extremely low rates of sperm retrieval on biopsy, compared to deletion of other gene sites which holds better prognosis of finding sperms on biopsy (e.g. AZF c).

Pearl of wisdom

- *Though pricey, genetic testing remains crucial in selected circumstances specially when transmission of genetic aberrations to off springs needs to be avoided.*

- *Genetic tests include Y-chromosome screening that evaluates integrity and identifies Y-chromosome micro-deletions (Or damages), karyotype test that evaluates the number of chromosomes e.g. Klinefelter syndrome (47XXY).*

V

Management of Male Factor Infertility

Treatment of male infertility aims to deliver greater numbers of healthy sperms and enabling them to be carried into the semen to fulfill competently their desired goal of fertilization. Fertility specialist will offer an ample therapeutic plan including life style modification, medical therapy, surgical interventions, referral to assisted reproduction clinics for sperm banking and application of various artificial reproductive techniques and finally offering psychological counseling.

Life Style Modification

As previously mentioned, many risk factors can affect male reproduction; this could explain the elevated and alarming worldwide trends of reduced male fecundity. Living healthy not only improves overall quality of life, but also offers significant improvements to the sperm forming machinery in the testis and testosterone production. It is highly recommended that your infertility specialist explores your lifestyle behaviors and search for any hazardous exposures that might explain fertility suppression. Quitting smoking is proven to be a highly appropriate measure to improve fertility and prevent the inadvertently reduced sperm counts. Additionally alcohol as described earlier is incriminated to cause sperm damage and hormonal disruption as consequence of its deleterious effect on the liver, same as with obesity which causes estrogen levels to rise counteracting the desired effects of testosterone, increased exposure to heat and radio frequency waves are well studied hazards that are linked to various sperm abnormalities, malnutrition and unhealthy diet render a person deficient in valuable vitamins and minerals essential for sperm formation, certain exposures e.g. chemicals, pesticides should be avoided, and finally the use of anabolic steroids for recreational purposes has to be immediately ceased for it is a known male contraceptive. Managing those risk factors requires determination and effort, however the significant benefits outweigh the trouble of eliminating them. Healthy diet remains one important aspect of a healthy life style and hence abiding to adequate intake of well-balanced meals including meat, greenery and fruits will supply you with enough antioxidants and nutrients that can restore many functional sperm defects. Stress can affect the whole body functions and needless to say human reproduction. During periods of stress testosterone production is affected implicating reduced sperm counts and fertility suppression.

Pearl of wisdom:

- *Life style modification is crucial, mandatory and most importantly beneficial, and though implementing control over your life style can impose real burden and requires much patience and perseverance, especially when many risk factors coexist, yet it is critical time to let healthy behaviors become a habit.*

Medical Therapy for Hormonal Imbalance

Conditions associated with low GN's:

This disorder is attributed to dysfunction of the brain glands (Pituitary and hypothalamus) caused by a variety of diseases of either congenital or acquired nature. The end result is failure of the brain glands to secrete the messenger hormones i.e. the gonadotropins (GN's), ultimately no signals are transmitted to the testis, leading to reduced testosterone secretion and suppressed sperm formation; implicating infertility. Congenital disorders are managed by hormone replacement therapy, given in the form of injections and are usually given for life. Injections should constitute both types of missing hormones, LH and FSH. LH aims to stimulate the testis to secret testosterone, while FSH promotes the process of sperm formation. In congenital conditions, affected children may present with delayed puberty and therefore therapy is commenced as early as the time of puberty. However in acquired cases, therapy aims to restore the brain gland's function, and hence to recommence LH and FSH secretion. This therapy is available, convenient, easy to administer. If this form of therapy fails, external substitution of the deficient hormones is initiated.

Pearl of wisdom:

- *Typically patients with low GN's present with low testosterone measurements and reduced sperm counts.*
- *Infertility specialist may request brain imaging e.g. MRI, to rule out any structural abnormalities causing suppression and damage of the brain glands.*
- *Anabolic steroids can result in shut down to the brain glands and ultimately significantly lowering LH and FSH levels.*

Conditions associated with high GN's:

This condition is characterized by failure of the testis to perform any of its designated functions namely testosterone secretion and/or sperm formation. As a result, the brain glands will sense this shortcoming and will attempt to resolve it by releasing higher levels of GN's (LH-FSH) aiming to uphold the testis, which is at risk of failure. Such patients present with high GN's and low testosterone levels and reduced sperm counts. Causes behind this disorder are conditions that cause progressive testicular dysfunction and ultimately failure e.g. testicular infections, chemotherapy, radiation therapy, severe trauma, ig-nored undescended testes, etc. Treatment involves managing all insults inflicting the testis as early as possible before irreversible damage ensues. Genetic disorders e.g. Klinefelter syndrome are incurable, since they are usually associated with severe atrophy and damage to the testis. Managing such condition is very delicate, and includes substituting the male with androgens (Testosterone) but only after offering early trials of sperm harvesting procedures (Read below). In the context of testicular failure, androgen therapy is usually given for life (In the form of exogenous testosterone shots). Injections should only be administered *after confirming testicular failure and complete incapacity of the testis to secret testosterone, and producing sperms (since exogenous testosterone administration will suppress any pre-existing sperm formation).* In situations where low testosterone is associated with elevated estradiol levels e.g. Klinefelter syndrome, your physician will prescribe anti estrogen therapy, which blocks the transformation of testosterone to estradiol, this form of therapy will result in elevation of testosterone and drop of estradiol to normal levels. At some point your physician will offer a testicular biopsy aiming to harvest sperms from the testis, and store them for future use through artificial reproductive techniques (Read below).

Pearl of wisdom:

- *Testicular failure is a serious condition, it may present with progressive diminution of sperm counts reaching in more severe cases a total absence of sperms in the ejaculate (A condition called 'Non-obstructive azoospermia'), hence it is highly advised to consider sperm banking when counts are progressively declining (Read below).*
- *Patients scheduled for chemotherapy and/or radiation therapy for diverse body cancers are highly advised to bank sperms prior to starting treatment since return of sperm formation after discontinuation of therapy is unpredictable (chemotherapy and radiation therapy are highly noxious to sperms and during therapeutic period sperm counts can reach very low and undetectable levels).*

High levels of Prolactin hormone:

As mentioned earlier, elevated prolactin levels can have detrimental effects on male reproduction, namely, suppression of GN's (LH–FSH) resulting in reduction of testosterone levels and suppression of sperm formation. Once diagnosed, your physician will rule out a possibility of medications adverse event, and will then evaluate your brain for possible structural abnormalities within the pituitary gland. Therapy includes medical and possibly surgical treatments. Medical therapy is a convenient approach, using commonly available medications. Oral therapy is usually given for a prolonged period of time until normalization of prolactin levels. In a more serious setting, a Prolactinoma should be ruled out (benign tumor of the pituitary gland). Small Prolactinoma may be treated medically, however it is always advisable to seek a neurosurgical evaluation since associated symptoms caused by compression of the lesion on adjacent vital structures may co-exist e.g. visual disturbance, and hence surgical removal may represent a valid option.

Pearl of wisdom:

- *Male factor infertility associated with headaches, visual disturbance, and any other neurological sings and symptoms may represent a Prolactinoma, which mandates a neurological evaluation.*

Treatment of Varicoceles

Management of varicoceles is still controversial, yet surgical treatment remains the primary option available. Whenever diagnosed with varicocele (whether after clinical or an ultrasound testing) the physician will determine the necessity of therapy according to the degree of disease. Usually varicoceles are staged based on their degree, and there are various ways of classification. Varicoceles are associated with progressive testicular damage, implicating progressive fertility suppression, yet not much evidence supports the benefit of treatment of varicoceles in infertile patients with normal semen parameters, or in patients with low grade varicocele. Varicocele repair may be indicated in the context of abnormal sperm test, palpable dilated veins and unexplained infertility. Surgical treatment of varicocele has many approaches, yet open surgery is commonly offered. However based on the current guidelines, your physician may propose microsurgical treatment. Microsurgery has recently been introduced into the field of urology and offers highly successful results. Using the magnification power of the surgical microscope the veins are more accurately visualized and easily controlled, while other vital structures are carefully preserved including the arteries and lymphatics (Lymphatics are vascular channels draining fluids from the testis and hence their inadvertent ligation may lead to a condition called 'Hydrocele' which is collection of watery fluid around the testis).

Pearl of wisdom:

- *According to some studies, when fertility is concerned, correction of varicocele may improve sperm DNA condition and reverse spermatic abnormalities.*
- *Discuss with your physician other alternatives to microsurgery used to treat of varicocele like open surgery, and laparoscopy.*
- *Embolization is an outpatient procedure and is an alternative option to surgery (yet offers less success rates compared to surgery), where the radiologist injects tiny particles through your veins (under X-ray guidance) leading to blockage of the varicocele veins.*

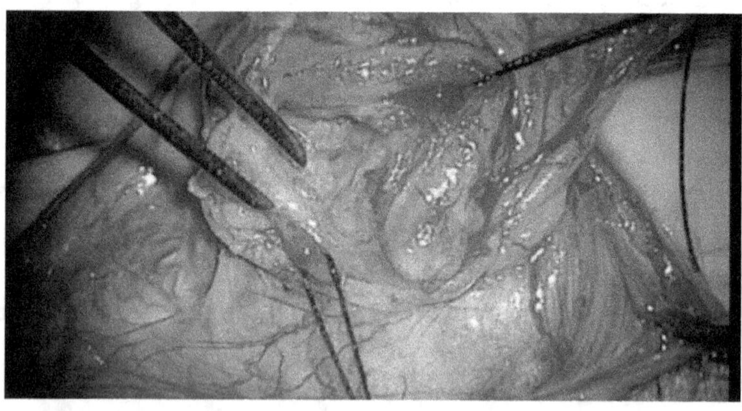

Microsurgical treatment of varicocele

Treatment of Low Sperm Counts (Oligozoospermia)

This condition is defined as reduced sperm counts (low concentration) below the internationally defined thresholds. According to the 2015 'WHO' reference ranges of semen parameters, a normal sperm concentration is at least 15 millions per each milliliter of semen. Numbers below the threshold of 15 millions/ml does not necessary imply absolute infertility, and chance of natural conception remains possible (*Though pregnancy rates are much lower than normal*). Many sperms are usually lost during their journey from the male to the female genital tract marching towards the ovum and undergoing fertilization; accordingly more favorable pregnancy rates are achieved with higher sperm concentrations (i.e., more number of sperms in each milliliter of semen). This condition may be associated with other abnormal seminal parameters including abnormally reduced sperm motility and increased shape aberrations (Collectively known as oligo-astheno-terato-zoospermia or referred to as OAT syndrome). This condition may result in delayed conception, sub-fertility, recurrent miscarriages, and total infertility (Because of dysfunctional sperms). Your infertility specialist will investigate and treat all possible causes behind such sperm anomalies, e.g. varicoceles, low testosterone levels or associated testicular infections. *If count continues to drop progressively, your infertility specialist may propose sperm banking (Freezing).* Storing sperms using banking is a very rational and convenient decision, since in some unfortunate situations; sperm counts may continue to decline reaching undetectable levels, and therefore having an adequate number of sperms stored minimizes the catastrophic agony of such context (Read below about sperm banking).

Pearl of wisdom:

- *Anomalies in semen parameters may frequently exist in men on their first sperm test, this however doesn't imply a true abnormality, since sperm counts may vary from one test to the other, so be advised to repeat the test prior to deciding on any further steps.*
- *Consider sperm banking when sperm counts are progressively declining; this is a tremendously crucial and wise decision.*

Treatment of Absence of Sperms in the ejaculate (Azoospermia)

Azoospermia is defined as absence of sperms in the ejaculate (the seminal liquid may still appear normal, yet is devoid from sperms). This can result from complete failure of sperm production in the testis, or presence of an obstruction along the sperm pathways; consequently hindering sperm passage. Differentiation between both types is crucial as each has a different treatment strategy. A common *yet inconclusive way* of differentiation is measuring the size of the testis. Dysfunctional testis tends to be smaller compared to a normally functioning testis (malfunctioning testis has less active and healthy tissues within), and since the obstructed testes may still function properly, they usually present with normal size. Ultimately by simply measuring the size of the testis one can predict the functional status and therefore make the difference between obstruction and dysfunction *(exceptions for this rule do exist where size is not a truly reliable method and biopsy is the only way to differentiate between both conditions).*

Non-Obstructive Azoospermia:

This condition refers to failure of the testes to produce sperms, and despite the apparent normal volume of the ejaculate, sperms are absent. *It is not uncommon that non-obstructive azoospermia is associated with severe testosterone hormone deficiency i.e. complete testicular failure* (Where both testicular functions are defective). This condition though rare but is considerably serious, and often leads to tremendous anxiety among inflicted patients. Non-obstructive azoospermia can be a congenital infliction or can develop later in life. Congenital causes are usually of genetic origin e.g. Y-chromosome micro-deletion and Kline-felter syndrome (Read earlier). Acquired causes include but are not limited to post exogenous androgen administration (Testosterone or T-shots or also referred to as anabolic steroids), undescended testes (Read earlier), chemotherapy, radiation therapy, Mumps Orchitis, etc. Non-obstructive azoospermia usually presents with variable degree of testicular size reduction reaching complete shrinkage in more severe cases, and is occasionally associated with signs and symptoms of testosterone hormone deficiency. Once diagnosed with non-obstructive azoospermia, your male infertility specialist will correct any associated disorders e.g. infections, hormonal imbalance or varicocele (There is limited evidence that correction of varicocele may reverse azoospermia and improve sperm production). Once the nocuous factors are corrected, the patient will be asked once again to give a semen sample for testing (Occasionally with hormonal treatment sperms may appear in the ejaculate). If no sperms were detected, your physician will discuss the next step that is usually a testicular biopsy and trial of sperm harvesting. Evidence suggests that some areas within the dysfunctional testis may still be functioning i.e. still producing sperms, yet in a limited capacity that doesn't enable those few sperms to appear into the ejaculate, and here lies the rational behind testicular biopsy in the context of non-obstructive azoospermia (Read below about sperm harvesting procedures).

Pearl of wisdom:

- *This might be the most valuable advice in the management of male infertility; at any point of time, before and after medical treatment, and whenever requested to perform a semen test, be advised to perform the test at a facility that can freeze and hence store any identified sperms, since occasionally few sperms are detected in the ejaculate, and once those sperms are luckily stored, they can be used in artificial reproduction (Read below about artificial reproductive techniques).*
- *Be informed that nowadays and with the help of advanced medical progress in sperm harvesting and the evolving artificial reproductive technology, many patients with non-obstructive azoospermia can father children, so be optimistic and don't lose hope.*

Obstructive Azoospermia:

Absence of sperms in the ejaculate can be attributed to obstruction at any level of sperm pathway and causes may include:

- Congenital (Genetic) absence of the vas deferens
- Occlusion of the vas deferens following various surgical procedures e.g. hernia repair
- Presence of abnormal lesions called 'Cysts' that block the flow of semen from the ejaculatory ducts into the urethra
- Ejaculatory duct obstruction
- Recurrent sexually transmitted infections that cause scar-

ring of the small sperm channels in the testis and epididy-mus and ultimately complete blockage of sperm pathways

Remember that obstruction is not equivalent to testicular fail-ure, and prognosis is generally favorable compared to non-obstructive azoospermia. Once diagnosed, your physician will try to locate the site of obstruction. Trans-rectal ultrasound (An ultrasound that is performed through the rectum) may be requested to better visualize the reproductive glands (For possible presence of cysts or ejaculatory ducts obstruction). Genetic testing (For both partners) is crucial to rule out the possibility of genetic mutation (CFTR gene mutation) in cases of congenital absence of the vas deferens (Read earlier). Pa-tients who have previously performed a vasectomy procedure (Surgically blocking the vas deferens on both sides as a male contraceptive technique) may be offered surgical reconstruction (Also referred to as refertilization surgery), however if not feasible, patient may elect to perform a testicular biopsy and use the retrieved sperms in artificial reproduction.

Pearl of wisdom:

- *Be aware that recurrent sexually transmitted diseases can even-tually cause obstruction to sperm pathways and unfortunately resulting in infertility.*
- *Obstruction of sperm pathways can still be associated with normal testicular function and normal sperm formation.*
- *Be advised that if surgical correction of obstruction is problem-atic, testis biopsy can be easily performed and harvested sperms are subsequently used in artificial reproduction.*

Treatment of Ejaculatory Disorders

Patients who have undergone pelvic, rectal or colonic operations, or had to surgically remove metastatic testicular cancers (tumors spread beyond the testis into the abdomen) and therefore are suspected to have some degree of damaged to their ejaculatory nerves, and may complain of dysfunctional ejaculation. To diagnose retrograde ejaculation (i.e. passage of semen into the urinary bladder instead of being ejected to the exterior) the patient is advised to perform a urine sample after ejaculating (Also referred to as post-ejaculatory urine analysis) to confirm the presence of sperms in the urine. Whenever no structural anomalies coexist (e.g. after prostate operations) several medical treatments can be used to restore ejaculation, ultimately the scheduled use of those medications at days of partner's ovulation will enable the male to ejaculate normally in to the vagina at times of highest fertility potential. Rapid ejaculation could be easily managed nowadays with a specifically designed on-demand medications that delay ejaculation for significant amount of time, these medications are safe and readily available, however, are listed as controlled-medications, hence, can not be taken without medical supervision and a prescription. On the other hand, delayed ejaculation could be managed through several ways including, psychological counseling and limiting certain behaviors like masturbation and use of pornography, which makes the act of sexual intercourse less arousing and less desirable, and hence leading to delayed ejaculation. However, in the most severe neurogenic conditions, where sensation is affected, like in diabetes or neurogenic diseases, the use of an intense penile-vibrators can assist the patient attain significant stimulation and hence climax and ejaculation.

Pearl of wisdom:

- *In retrograde ejaculation, sperms can be easily retrieved from the urine, and are prepared for use through assisted reproduction (after applying specific form of treatment to the sperms).*
- *Simple testicular biopsy is another convenient option in the context of ejaculatory dysfunction (to harvest sperms directly from the testis and use them in assisted reproduction).*
- *For patients who had previous vasectomy operation, reversal procedures are commonly performed using microsurgery, and fortunately offers favorable success rates.*
- *Concerning patients on alpha-blocker therapy for enlarged prostates, be advised to consult your urologist to hold therapy during the period of your partner's ovulation to restore normal ejaculation*
- *Share with your physician your list of medications, since delayed ejaculation could actually be side effect of certain drugs.*

Role of Supplements in Male Infertility

Nutritional supplements have gained significant popularity over the last decade, possibly because of increased population awareness and focus of the research community on studying various alternative resources and remedies to treat male infertility. Though no definite universal guidelines are currently available for practitioners, many reports have shown possible improvement of sperm parameters after incorporation of supplements into the management of male infertility. There are many nutritional additives obtainable from the market, and are either available as single agents or a combination of supplements packed all together in a form of pill or a dissolvable powder. Sperm formation is a critical process requiring a delicately healthy micro-environment, and achieving this requires maintaining low levels of 'Free Oxygen Radicals' also know as 'reactive oxygen species or ROS', such particles are normally produced by the sperms or simply infiltrating from other sources, they serve to perform several spermatic functions, however their excess can be detrimental on sperm DNA integrity and ultimately fertility. Fortunately the naturally occurring antioxidants act against the over production of ROS and counteract their harmful effects. Occasionally disharmony of this sensitive balance may take place (consistent with reduced antioxidant protective function in face of deliberate rise in ROS production), implicating major damage to the sperm DNA. Consequently many generations of sperms with defective DNA and weak fertilizing capacity are on the front line. Studies show that increased ROS secretion is linked to several conditions e.g. smoking, exposure to industrial chemicals and pesticides, heat, irradiation, varicocele, inflammation, fever, strenuous exercise, infection, trauma, etc. The concept behind incorporating antioxidant supplements in the management of male infertility is to overcome the deleterious effects of elevated ROS levels, offering more stability to the sperm DNA and ultimately amelioration of sperm function. Only the most common supplements with highest clinical significance will be discussed here (*Caution: This is not a prescription and you should consult your physician prior to starting any medication or food supplement to avoid any detrimental effects*).

Coenzyme Q10 (Co-Q10), is a vitamin like molecule, capable of producing significant amounts of energy within the cells, and is therefore commonly found in organs with high energy requirement. Many studies suggest that Co-Q10 could improve sperm parameters including concentration and motility. This explains the high trends of using CO-Q10 as a supplemental agent in the management of male infertility. Natural sources include whole grain, cabbage, carrots, onion, spinach and nuts.

Carnitine, an important substance that is present in many cells of our body, it plays an important role in the process of energy production. It also acts as antioxidant protecting the cells from the damaging effects of ROS. Carnitine has been shown to promote semen parameters including improvement in numbers, motility potential and ameliorates viability of the sperms. Natural sources include meat products e.g. red meat, fish and poultry, with scant concentrations in vegetables and fruits.

Selenium, a molecule with high antioxidant property, it reduces the deleterious effects of the ROS. Additionally, selenium plays an important role in maintaining the integrity of sperm formation. When combined with other supplement e.g. vitamin E, selenium may offer better antioxidant property. Natural sources include nuts, fish, meat, egg, garlic and cereals.

Zinc is an important molecule that supports the actions of many enzymes; it is also essential for DNA integrity, stability of the immune system and testosterone formation (*Hence, Zinc deficiency may lead to reduced testosterone levels*). Zinc has an antioxidant capacity, offers protection against ROS and reduces DNA damage. Natural sources include crab, lobster, red meat, wheat, spinach, pumpkin and squash seeds, cashew nuts, cocoa and chocolate, beans and mushrooms.

Vitamins A, C and E are potent antioxidants, neutralizing the effects of ROS and hence offer support to various sperm functions. Vitamin C protects against sperm DNA damage. Natural sources of vitamin A and C include fruits, vegetables where raw seeds, almonds and spinach are rich in vitamin E.

Phytoestrogens, which are plant derived chemical substances, occasionally marketed as food supplements. These substances resemble the structure of estrogen molecule (a female reproductive hormone), and thus when administered into males they may behave as estrogen and may possibly interfere with the hormonal balance responsible for reproduction and normal development. Phytoestrogens are found in soybeans, soy products and flax seeds. The effect of phytoestrogen on male fertility is still unclear, yet several conflicting studies have shown negative effect on male reproduction and semen parameters

Pearl of wisdom:

- *Food supplement is an important tool used in the management of male infertility, yet no current guidelines have demonstrated a standardization to their use.*
- *Consult your health care provider before using nutritional supplements to protect against potential adverse effects.*
- *Study the mode of the administration of each supplement as they may differ in relation to the time of the day and their relation to the meals.*
- *The ideal food supplement is a well balanced diet.*

Sperm Harvesting Procedures (Testicular Biopsy)

Also referred to as testicular biopsy or sperm retrieval procedure. It is the process by which the surgeon will surgically remove tiny parts from your testis and examine under a microscope for presence of sperms. Such procedures are better performed at a facility that can store sperms i.e. reproductive lab. Whenever a patient is diagnosed with azoospermia (Complete absence of sperms), one crucial question is proposed '*Is it an Obstructive or Non-Obstructive Azoospermia?*' *(Read earlier for definitions)*

Despite the different clinical parameters guiding the clinician to make the right diagnosis, there remain situations where clinical judgment is insufficient and hence biopsy becomes imperative.

Performing a testicular biopsy offers many benefits including in the first place an accurate mean of differentiation between obstruction and non-obstruction (Normal sperm formation exists in the context of obstruction and not in non-obstructive azoospermia) and secondly the possibility of retrieving sperms in non-obstructive azoospermia patients, hence storing and using them in artificial reproduction.

Before performing a testicular biopsy discuss with your in-fertility specialist the timing at which your partner will get prepared for assisted reproduction, or ART (Read later on different forms of ART's) , some reproductive endocrinologists prepare the female partner only after sperms are successfully retrieved (i.e. Freezing and storing any identified sperms and subsequently using them at a different time frame) to avoid unnecessary female hormonal manipulation in the unfortunate event of not finding sperms on biopsy, however others believe that yield of sperms from biopsy is commonly scant, and since during the process of sperm storage (Which includes freezing and thawing) some of those successfully retrieved sperms (Which are commonly fragile) can get damaged, so it is preferable to have the female partner ready at the same day of biopsy and immediately using any identified sperms (Freshly retrieved) without the need for storing them (By freezing). On the other way round, the cost of such rationale is the futile female hormonal preparation in the event of not finding sperms on biopsy.

Different techniques of testicular biopsy are currently available and each is offered depending on the different clinical context.

Needle aspiration, *also known as Testicular Sperm Aspiration (or TESA)*

This is the simplest form of testicular biopsy, done as an out patient procedure. It is performed using a needle that is connected to a syringe for aspiration, the surgeon will initially inject small dose of local anesthetic into the skin overlying the testis (Usually a preference is given to the larger testis) and when the skin gets numb, the surgeon will insert the needle directly into the testis, and while the syringe is on the aspiration mode, tissues from within the testis are sucked through the needle. Tissue fragments aspirated from the testis are then pulled and collected in specific tubes for analysis. This is usually done at a facility where immediate examination of the tissues is possible. If sperms are identified, the surgeon will stop aspiration. Advantages of this procedure include being convenient (Office based and under local anesthesia), low cost, not time consuming and not requiring significant expertise. Disadvantages include being random (Inability to visually identify, choose and select viable and apparently healthy testicular fragments for analysis), rate of successful sperm retrieval is low, and is possibly traumatic (Bleeding may occur after repeated passage of the needle into the testis). TESA is commonly indicated when obstruction is suspected and sperm formation is maintained, and hence sticking a needle anywhere into the testis will presumably yield large numbers of sperms.

Open testicular biopsy, *also referred to as Testicular Sperm Extraction (TESE)*

Surgical removal of small fragments from the testis under local anesthesia. The surgeon will cut through the scrotal skin and the testis exposing underlying testicular tissues and small pieces are surgically removed. Tissues are then sent to the lab for examination, and when sperms are identified they are used by assisted reproduction e.g. IVF or ICSI (read below). TESE shares with needle aspiration the same advantages of being convenient, quick, moderately inexpensive and doesn't require much expertise, yet in addition to this, it offers better sperm retrieval rates (compared to TESA) as more tissue volumes are examined. On the other hand it lacks accuracy, since testicular tissues are significantly small and assessing their quality by the naked eye remains a difficult task, therefore it is mostly arbitrary when it comes to selecting tissues for analysis.

Micro-Dissection Testicular Sperm Extraction, *also referred to as Micro-dissection TESE or MTESE.*

This modern technique offers better results and fewer complications. Recently microsurgery has been introduced into the field of urology (using the operating microscope which magnifies up to 25 times), and has helped trained urologists to better visualize the seminiferous tubules of the testis. MTESE is a surgical procedure that involves opening the testis (more widely compared to TESE) and using the magnification offered by the surgical microscope, the seminiferous tubules are carefully studied. The surgeon will search for and retrieve the best-looking and healthiest tissues avoiding the removal of unnecessary testicular fragments and hence preserving the volume of the testis. Retrieved tissues are then sent for analysis and exploration for presence of sperms to be used ultimately by assisted reproduction. This technique may result in higher success rates compared to other forms of testicular biopsy. Improved results are attributed to the magnification power offered by the surgical microscope that significantly improved sperm retrieval rates. On the other hand it added a burden of increased surgical time, higher cost of procedure and mandatory expertise of the treating surgeon (microsurgical training).

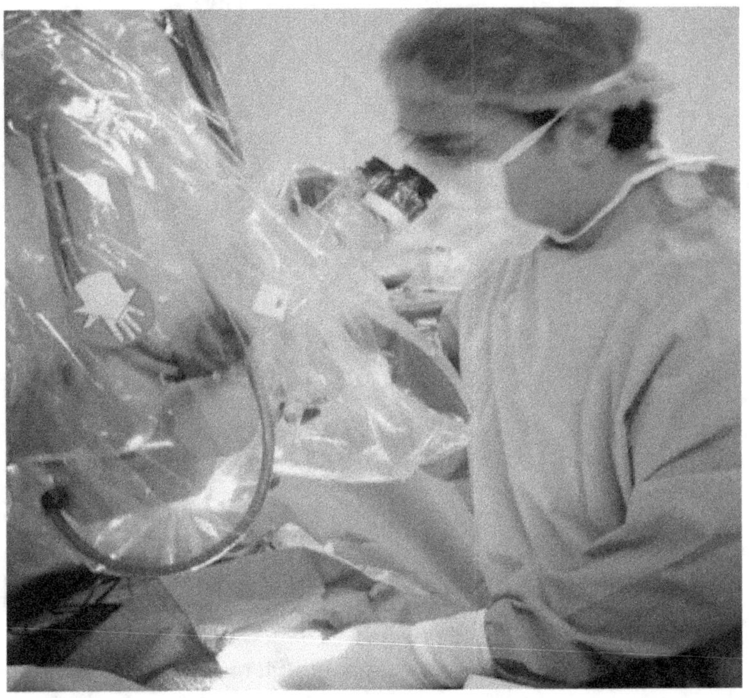

Undergoing Micro–Dissection Testicular Sperm Extraction.

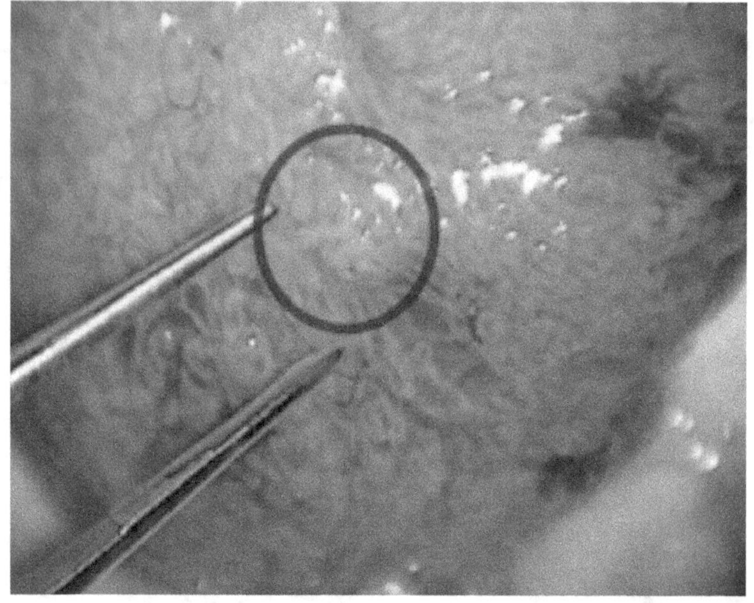

***Magnified image under the microscope showing
sperm-harboring potential areas.***

Testicular mapping:

Testicular mapping combination of the previous, where the surgeon performs multiple testicular aspirations (TESA) at different levels, and assigning a number to each zone tested, and if sperms are identified, the surgeon will perform a micro-dissection TESE on the same zone that is declared to contain sperms.

Pearl of wisdom:

- *The infertility specialist will educate you on different forms of testicular biopsy and will elect to choose what suites your condition better.*

- *Don't forget to perform a semen test prior to biopsy since occasionally some sperms may be found in the ejaculate and accordingly biopsy becomes optional.*
- *TESA and TESE are better reserved for patients with obstruction and hence the likelihood of finding sperms is high. Sometimes the yield of sperms from biopsy is scant and multiple biopsies are required.*
- *Absence of sperms on the first biopsy doesn't exclude the possibility of finding sperms on future repeat biopsies; so don't lose hope.*
- *Remember that MTESE offers higher sperm retrieval rates.*
- *Biopsy results are more favorable when male reproductive hormones are maintained within normal ranges for stable period of time; so always check hormones before biopsy.*
- *Don't perform a testicular biopsy while under anticoagulation therapy (blood thinning therapy for prevention of strokes and vascular diseases), it may result in large blood collection in your scrotum after the procedure.*
- *In some cases your testosterone level may decline transiently after biopsy.*

Assisted Reproduction - Artificial Reproductive Techniques (ART)

This modern and advanced field of medicine has lead to endless success stories, and has gained an overwhelming reputation worldwide. It is defined as the medical techniques that assist patients suffering from infertility to achieve pregnancy. It includes several techniques but in principle this technology bypasses sexual intercourse as a method for fertilization, and depending on the condition; assisted reproduction can overcome defects encountered at any phase of natural conception. To understand what assisted reproduction offers, we first have to go through the journey of the sperm and the ovum.

The journey starts when the baby sperms (Immotile) mature inside the testis (Hence become motile), then those millions of mature sperms will travel through the male ducts reaching the storage glands. At this point, sperms will receive the nourishment that will support them during their enduring journey (Which is long, critical and tough journey). The nourishing secretions come from the seminal vesicle and the prostate gland at time of ejaculation. In the vagina the sperms will struggle enduring a hostile milieu compared to that of the male genital tract (High level of acidity that is actually hazardous to sperms). Fortunately the accompanying secretions from the seminal vesicle and prostate gland will help overcome this obstacle. Ultimately numerous sperms will die by the moment they enter the vagina (That's why higher number of sperms are required since many will be lost during their journey). The remaining sperms escaping the acidity massacre will then ascend to the uterus through the cervix helped by the sticky cervical secretions that act like pathways through which sperms will travel, however at this stage many sperms will get attacked and unfortunately killed by the great numbers of existing immunity cells (As sperms being recognized as invaders). The remaining sperms continue their marathon from the uterus towards the fallopian tube that is considered a heavenly place for them. In the fallopian tube, the environment is less hostile than before, however the number of sperms remaining have become significantly lower compared to the number initially ejaculated into the vagina (As by then greater number of sperms are already lost). Mid way through the fallopian tube, the ovum will be waiting for the fittest sperm that successfully managed to overcome all previous obstacles and is ready to undergo fertilization. When the first sperm penetrates the walls of the ovum, no other sperm is allowed to enter afterwards. The united sperm and ovum are by now called an embryo, which will start to grow one cell after the other while being pushed by the fallopian tube towards the uterus. When reaching the uterine cavity, the embryo will get buried deep into its layers like a seed buried into the soil. By then the source of nourishment to the newly formed embryo is from the layers of the uterus surrounding the embryo.

Intra-Uterine Insemination (IUI):

Whenever sperm counts are low (Oligozoospermia) the couple may be offered to perform an IUI. This procedure is performed by injecting the seminal fluid (the liquid containing sperms) near the period of ovulation into the uterus, aiming to bypass the obstacles faced by the sperms in the vagina and in some cases the cervix. This technique offers many benefits especially when sperm counts are low. With IUI the sperm journey is shorter and greater number of sperms reach the ovum, and therefore the chance of conception is improved.

In-Vitro Fertilization (IVF):

When sperm counts are significantly low, the couple may elect to a more sophisticated form of assisted reproduction. The female is given medications to facilitate ovulation; this will stimulate the ovary to release more than one ovum. Ultimately those ova are retrieved by the gynecologist and are prepared in the lab for assisted reproduction. At this point, the partner's sperms are examined in the lab and the best quality sperms are collected and mixed with the retrieved ova in specific forms of dishes (Sperms are added to the same dish where the ovum is stored). The whole specimen is left aside for a period of time under constant monitoring (waiting for a potent sperm to penetrate the ovum and hence fertilizes it). After couple of days, the specimen is re-checked for fertilization, and if results are favorable for successful fertilization, the whole specimen is re-introduced into the uterus hoping for appropriate implantation. Then the female is monitored using serial pregnancy tests to confirm or refute pregnancy.

Intra-Cytoplasmic Sperm Injection (ICSI):

In more severe cases of male infertility, where only scant number of sperms are offered (e.g. after micro-dissection TESE for non-obstructive azoospermia patients) ICSI becomes indicated. In this technique, again the ova are retrieved from the ovaries and the sperms are collected, and using a very tiny instruments and a complex microscope, the best offered sperm is injected delicately into the ovum (hence the name 'Intra-cytoplasmic sperm injection'). The specimen is monitored for couple of days and if fertilization occurred, what is now called an 'embryo' is transferred into the uterus and the patient is followed with serial pregnancy tests to confirm or refute pregnancy.

Pearl of wisdom:

- *The female infertility specialist (Reproductive endocrinologist) plays a pivotal role deciding which assisted reproductive technique better suites the couple.*
- *Choosing between assisted reproductive techniques depends on different parameters out of which are the duration of infertility, sperm count, sperm DNA condition, age of the female partner and the financial burden of each technique.*
- *Prior to various assisted reproductive techniques, the female partner will be prepared using a medical treatment that manipulates her reproductive hormones; therefore a thorough discussion ensuring proper comprehension of the consequences and implications of hormonal manipulations should be implemented.*
- *Whenever scheduled for an appointment with a reproductive endocrinologist, it is important to convey your inquiries (if present) about the credibility, privacy and success rates related*

to the affiliated center where the procedure is going to take place.

- If you already have sperms stored (Banked), be advised to give a fresh sample on the day of the procedure and if sperms are identified, you may elect to use them rather than relying on the stored ones (keep the stored sperms for future needs).
- In unfortunate situations, assisted reproduction may fail, and despite the agony of this outcome, be patient and don't lose hope, chances of success are always promising with future cycles.

VI

The Final Pearl

Wrap It Up

Male Infertility is on the rise, increasing in incidence day after day, possibly because of the wide range of hazardous exposures frequently encountered in our so-called 'modern life style'.

Having this well said, medical care concerned with the study and management of male infertility have recently evolved, successfully offering new guidelines, remedies and most importantly hope to the males previously entitled sterile.

Delay in pregnancy is not a synonym of infertility, and it is strongly advised to use the term 'Infertility' with caution.

As mentioned earlier in the chapters of this book, it may take a normal couple one year in an average to get a fruitful pregnancy, and hence patience in such context is the righteous virtue.

Consulting a male fertility specialist is the first step towards successful therapy, and delaying this step may result in detrimental effect on the plan of therapy.

Maintaining an appropriate communication between your fertility specialist and the reproductive lab is crucial when it comes to sperm banking in face of low sperm counts.

A healthy living, embraced by a well balanced diet, regular exercise, and avoiding of unnecessary hazardous exposures e.g. smoking and alcohol consumption, remains a very critical step in improving and/or maintaining male fertility and sexuality.

Hope remains the best remedy, one that is essential during the whole journey from sterility to fatherhood.

The male infertility research is running fast and everyday a new hope is born, so stay optimistic and don't lose hope.

At the end, it is critically important to understand that medical disorders are better dealt with by a qualified professional in person, and other means including this book, or online Internet readings should never replace the proper evaluation by a health care professional.

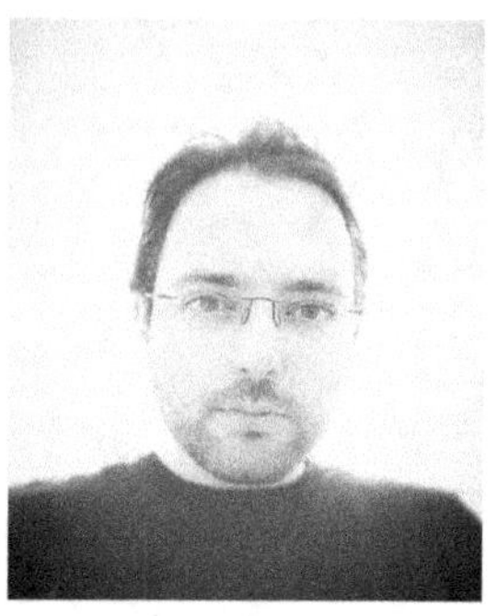

About the Author

Hussein Kandil, MD - Urologist graduated from the division of urology at Saint George Hospital University Medical Center (SGHUMC) in Beirut, Lebanon, and sub-specialized in andrology at the division of urology at the University of Illinois at Chicago (UIC), USA. Currently running a men's health and fertility division at *Fakih IVF Fertility Center* in UAE.

Andrology is the field of medicine that specializes in the medical and surgical management of males suffering from infertility and/or sexual dysfunction.

In his practice, Dr. Kandil sees male patients everyday, many of which are men having difficulty starting a family because of their infertility/sub-fertility and/or sexual disorders. With time, this helped attain a more profound understanding concerning men's health and its related disorders.

Being a professional, actively engaged in the field of human reproduction, it has become mandatory to come out with this comprehensive manual, guiding males suffering from infertility/sub-fertility which happens to be on the rise in our current time.

I hope you find in this book a pearl of wisdom, well embraced within its pages, one that will make your journey overcoming your fertility concerns less enduring and more successful, leaving no chance for ambiguity or misconception, resulting after all in a healthy male reproductive and overall well being.

You can connect with me on:

🌐 https://fakihivf.com/doctor/dr-hussein-kandil-mbbch-facs

Also by Dr. Hussein Kandil

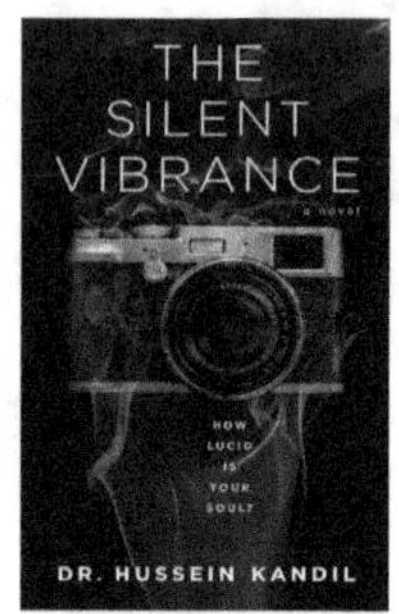

The Silent Vibrance: How Lucid Is Your Soul?

Gifted photographer, Eve Solace brightens hearts with the shadows in her pictures. The only heart she can't brighten is her own. Orphaned by a tragic fire, she is shy of confronting the world except through her lens. Things change when she encounters her first love, unearths mysterious messages from her past, and discovers a new way to understand the world through lucid dreaming. What follows is a series of experiences that connect Eve with her soul and empower her mind beyond her conscious grasp, or ours. In this fictional tale that reveals the potential of the mind and soul, physician Hussein Kandil takes us on a personal journey with Eve as she liberates herself through the gift of lucid dreaming, which in return allows her to escape her inner prison and empowers her to recapture long-lost relationships.

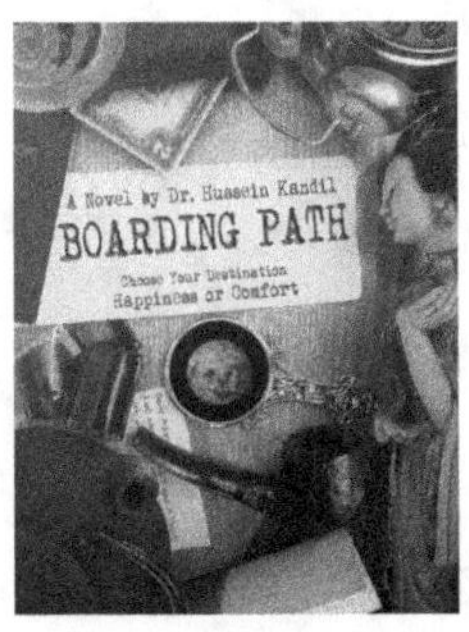

Boarding Path: Choose Your Destination 'Happiness or Comfort'?

Which path will you choose: happiness or comfort? These are the forces that have been plaguing Adam's soul. After years of devoutly serving his patients, a psychologist realizes that comfort and routine no longer satisfy his basic human needs. On a whim, Adam journeys to Japan in an effort to challenge his mundane habits only to find that all of humanity struggles with the same issues worldwide. While in Japan, he runs into a series of interesting characters that reshape his understanding of life, society, and human nature. He discovers that the solution to his and society's problems lies in answering one question: Which path to choose happiness or comfort?

www.ingramcontent.com/pod-product-compliance
Lightning Source LLC
Chambersburg PA
CBHW072253260726
48657CB00004BA/1584